An Essay on Hasheesh

Victor Robinson, M.D.

What is left for us modern men? We cannot be Greek now. The cypress of knowledge springs, and withers when it comes in sight of Troy; the cypress of pleasure likewise, if it has not died already at the root of cankering Calvinism; the cypress of religion is tottering. What is left? Science for those who are scientific. Art for artists, and all literary men are artists in a way. Bus science falls not to the lot of all. Art is hardly worth pursuing now. What is left? Hasheesh, I think: Hasheesh of one form or another. We can dull the pangs of the present by living the past again in reveries or learned studies, by illusions of the fancy and a self-indulgent dreaming. Take down the perfumed scrolls; open, unroll, peruse, digest, intoxicate your spirit with the flavor. Behold, here is the Athens of Plato in your narcotic visions; Buddha and his anchorites appear; the raptures of St. Francis and the fire-oblations of St. Dominic; the phantasms of mythologies; the birth-throes of religion, the neurotism of chivalry, the passion of past poems; all pass before you in your Maya world of hasheesh, which is criticism.

– JOHN ADDINGTON SYMONDS.

Robinson, Victor (1886–1947)
  An Essay on Hasheesh / by Victor Robinson, M.D. ;
  ISBN   1434808971
  EAN-13 9781434808974
edited by David M. Gross

10 9 8 7 6 5 4 3 2 1

Foreword

THE REQUEST FOR a second edition of *An Essay on Hasheesh*, revives memories of the first issue. This Essay was written in the spring of 1910, and two years later appeared in a medical journal, from which it was reprinted in book form (1912). In certain quarters, the fear was expressed that the Essay would be responsible for the formation of clubs of hasheesh-eaters, but on the whole the little volume found favor in literary and scientific circles: we recall our "picture in the papers," and that a score of reviewers hailed us as the American De Quincey. The Essay formed the basis of various editorials, we were invited to read it in medical schools, and it was quoted in such diverse sources as Professor H. L. Hollingsworth's *Psychological Aspects of Drug Action*, Mr. Max Eastman's *The Sense of Humor*, and Dr. Frank P. Davis' *Impotency, Sterility, and Artificial Impregnation*. The first edition was not large, and with the passing of time it reached the stage of "out of print." The call for the Essay, though seldom clamorous, has continued until the present, and recently, instead of diminishing, has rather increased.

Most writers welcome the opportunity to edit their work, to show what they have learned between editions, and we felt there was much we wished to revise in this dithyrambic production. We remembered we had put everything in this Essay, from prescriptions to poetry, and here is the chance to control the grandiloquence. Then there was that exuberant passage beginning, "He who conquers disease is greater than the builder of cities or the creator of empires," which so enraged Thomas G. Atkinson, of Chicago, that he wrote one of his finest editorials about it. We agree with the doctor, and if we were not so dilatory a correspondent we would have written to him long ago and told him so. Of course, we would now modify this extravagant paragraph, and bring it into proper focus. We even thought of substituting a new title, since the New York Evening Post had thus chided us: "Has not our love of conciseness carried us too far in the matter of book titles? What can one tell about the contents of a novel that is labelled *Peter and Jane*, or *The Casement*? How much information is conveyed by such phrases as *Health and Happiness*, or *An Essay on Hasheesh*?"

Accordingly, we regarded "second edition," as synonymous with "revised and enlarged edition," and for the first time in years we opened the Essay, blue-pencil in our now veteran hand. But a few moments with the Essay, and we realized that all thought of revision must be abandoned. When we wrote *An Essay on Hasheesh*, we lived in a different world, into which we could no longer enter. We seemed to be surveying the work of another, and though we could admire or condemn, we could not alter. Thus this second edition of the Essay is identical with the first. The uncurbed style, the pithy title, and even the passage which justly caused Dr. Atkinson to see red, are left unamended. In turning the following pages, the odor of the hemp-fields again teases our nostrils, but we can never recapture the mood in which we wrote this manuscript. We give it, therefore, to our readers, in its original form, as an expression of a lost rhapsodic period of our existence.

True are the words of Friedrich Rückert, master of thirty languages, poet and Orientalist, who revelled in the lands of hasheesh: "Youth, enthusiasm, and tenderness are like the days of spring. Instead of complaining, O my heart, of their brief duration, try to enjoy them."

V.R.
May 1925

An Essay on Hasheesh

An Essay on Hasheesh

"And now, borne far through the steaming air floats an odor, balsamic, startling; the odor of those plumes and stalks and blossoms from which is exuding freely the narcotic resin of the great nettle. The nostril expands quickly, the lungs swell out deeply to draw it in: fragrance once known in childhood, ever in the memory afterward, and able to bring back to the wanderer homesick thoughts of midsummer days in the shadowy, many-toned woods, over into which is blown the smell of the hemp-fields."

ALLEN: *The Reign of Law.*

"At the mere vestibule of the temple I could have sat and drunk in ecstasy forever, but lo! I am yet more blessed. On silent hinges the doors swing open, and I pass in."

LUDLOW: *The Hasheesh Eater.*

AILING MAN HAS ransacked the world to find balms to ease him of his pains. And this is only natural, for what doth it profit a man if he gain the whole world and lose his digestion? Let the tiniest nerve be but inflamed, and it will bend the proudest spirit: humble is a hero with a toothache! It is doubtful of Buddha himself could have maintained his equanimity with a bit of dust on his conjunctiva. Cæsar had a fever – and the eye that awed the world did lose its lustre, and the tongue that bade the Romans write his speeches in their books cried like a sick girl. Our flesh is heir to many ills, and alas when the heritage falls due. Even pride and prejudice are then forgotten, and Irishmen in need of purgatives are willing to use rhubarb grown on English soil, while the Foreign Colombo gathered by the feral natives in the untamed forests of Quilimani is consumed by ladies who never saw anything wilder than a Fabian Socialist.

The modern descendant of Hippocrates draws his Materia Medica from the uttermost ends of the earth: linseed from busy Holland and floretted marigold from the exotic Levant; cuckoo's cap from little Helvetia, and pepper-elder from ample Brazil; biting cubebs from spicy Borneo and fringed lichens from raw-winded Iceland; sweet flag from the ponds of Burmah, coto bark from the thickets of Bolivia, sleeping nightshade from the woods of Algeria, brownish rhatany from the sands of Peru, purple crocus from the pastures of Greece, aromatic vanilla from the groves of Mexico, golden seal from the retreats of Canada, knotty aleppo from the plains of Kirghiz, fever-tree from the hills of Tasmania, white saunders from the mountains of Macassar. Idols are broken daily nowadays, but the daughter of Æsculapius does not fear, for Hygeia knows she will always have a frenzied world of worshippers to kneel at her every shrine in every land.

All the reservoirs of nature have been tapped to yield medicines for man. From the mineral kingdom we take the alkali metals, the nitrogen group, the compounds of oxygen, the healing waters, the halogens, the nitrate of silver, the sulphate of copper, the carbonate of sodium, the chloride of mercury, the hydroxide of potassium, the acetate of lead, the citrate of lithium, the oxide of calcium, and the similar salts of half a hundred elements from Aluminum to Zincum.

From the vegetable kingdom we extract the potent alkaloid; all things that blossom and bloom, we knead them as we list: the broad rhizome of iris, the wrinkled root of lappa, the inspissated juice of aloes, the flower-heads of anthemis, the outer rind of orange, the inner bark of cinnamon, the thin arillode of macis, the dense sclerotium of ergot, the ovoid kernel of nutmeg, the pitted seed of rapa, the pale spores of club-moss, the spongy pith of sassafras, the bitter wood of quassia, the smoothish bark of juglans, the unripe fruit of hemlock, the fleshy bulb of scilla, the brittle leaves of senna, the velvet thallus of agaric, the balsamic resin of benzoin, the scaly strobiles of hops, the styles and stigmas of zea.

The animal kingdom has likewise been forced to bring tribute to its highest brother: we use in medicine the blood-sucking leech, the natural emulsion from the mammary glands of the cow, the internal fat from the abdomen of the hog, the coppery-green Spanish fly, the globular excrements of the leaping antelope, the fixed oil from the livers of the cod, the fresh bile of the stolid ox, the vitellus of the hen's egg, the fatty substance from the huge head of the sperm-whale, the odorous secretion of the musk-deer, the swimming-bladder of regal fish, the inner layer of the oyster-shell, the branched skeleton of the red polyp, the dried follicles of the boring beaver, the bony horns of the crimson deer, the thyroid glands of the simple sheep, the coagulated serum from the blood of the horse, the wax and honey from the hive of the busy bee, and even the disgusting cockroaches that infest the kitchen-shelves and climb all over the washtubs are used as a diuretic and for dropsy.

Little it matters by whom the healing agent was ushered in, for mankind in its frantic search for health asks not the creed or color of its medical savior: Pipsissewa was introduced into medicine by the redskins, buchu by the Hottentots, quassia by a negro slave, zinc valerianate by a French prince, krameria by a Spanish refugee, ipecac by the Brazilian aborigines, guaiac by a syphilitic warrior, aspidium by a Swiss widow.

"Medicine," wrote the greatest of literary physicians, "appropriates everything from every source that can be of the slightest use to anybody who is ailing in any way, or like to be ailing from any cause. It learned from a monk how to use antimony, from a Jesuit how to cure agues, from a friar how to cut for stone, from a soldier how to treat gout, from a sailor how to keep off scurvy, from a postmaster how to sound the Eustachian tube, from a dairy-maid how to prevent small-pox, and from an old market-woman how to catch the itch-insect. It borrowed acupuncture and the moxa from the Japanese heathen, and was taught the use of lobelia by the American savage."

And all these substances are daily being powdered, sifted, granulated, desiccated, percolated, macerated, distilled, sublimed, cominuted, dissolved, precipitated, filtered, strained, expressed, clarified, crystallized, ignited, fused, calcined, torrified and deflagrated into powders, pills, wafers, capsules, ampoules, extracts, tinctures, infusions, decoctions, syrups, cordials, essences, magmas, suppositories, tablets, troches, ointments, plasters, abstracts, liniments, collodions, cataplasms and so on and so on.

And all these finished preparations have a most laudable object in view – the eradication of disease and the alleviation of pain. Ah, this is indeed a quest worth the striving for! To accomplish the quadrature of the circle, or ferret out the secret of perpetual motion, may be highly interesting, though of problematical value only; but when a clammy sweat bathes the brow, and the delicate nerves twitch till the tortured human frame shakes in anguish, how important is it to be able to lift the veil from a condition like this! He who conquers disease is greater than the builder of cities or the creator of empires. His value is above the poets, statesmen cannot be compared unto him, educators equal him not in worth. A careful economist like John Stuart Mill tells us it is doubtful if all the labor-saving machinery ever invented has lessened for a single day the work of a single human being, – but when a discovery is made in medicine it becomes a sun which sheds its beneficence on all who suffer. The sick pauper of to-day lying in a charity hospital receives better medical treatment than the sick potentate of yesterday lying in his costly palace.

But so far medical science has only unhorsed, not overthrown, its ancient antagonist. In spite of all the remedies, in spite of all the research, mankind as yet possesses no satisfactory antidote for suffering; it knows no drug which can give pain its *congé* for more than a transient period.

But although the time of relief be limited, the simple fact that there are substances which do have some power over pain is sufficient to make the study of narcotism highly important. And of all the narcotics – a narcotic being roughly defined as a substance which relieves pain and produces excitability followed by sleep – none is more alluring to the imagination than the intoxicating hemp-plant, scientifically known as *Cannabis sativa* and popularly famed as hasheesh – those strange flowering-tops that appeal to a pot-bellied bushman of Australia who smokes it in a pipe of animal tusks, and to so hyper-esoteric a *littérateur* as Charles Baudelaire of the Celestial City of Art.

The habitat of the hemp-plant is extensive: not by the hand of man were the seeds sown that gave it birth near the Caspian Sea, where it wildly flourishes on the banks of the immense Volga – that might mass of liquid ever stupendously rolling through a limitless continent; it climbs the Altai range and thrives where the Himalaya rears its stony head ten thousand feet on high; it extends to Persia, and China knows it; the Congo river and the hot Zambesi bathe it in Africa, it is not a stranger in sunny France, and how well it thrives in Kentucky the numerous readers of the *Reign of Law* will ever remember.

In the seventeenth century Rumphius noticed that there were differences between the hemp grown in India and the hemp grown in Europe. In the nineteenth century Lamarck accepted these distinctions, and believing the Indian hemp to be a separate species, agreed in calling it *Cannabis indica* as a distinction from the *Cannabis sativa* of Linnæus and Willdenow. But it is now conceded that from a botanical standpoint the variations are by no means certain or important enough to warrant the maintenance of Indian hemp as a species distinct from common hemp. And as the greater includes the lesser, in botany as well as in geometry, its botanical name is *Cannabis sativa*, with *Cannabis indica* as one variety, just as *Cannabis americana* is another variety.

The hemp grown in Russia is of a fibrous quality, and is largely used for the galleys – to hang the opponents of despotism. In England many a bold highwayman has been embraced by it the last moment of his roving life, and has thus philanthropically given his mother-tongue a chance to enrich herself. For instance, a hempie means a rascal for whom the hemp grows, a hempen collar means the hangman's noose; a hempen widow means one whose husband has been hanged; to sow hemp means to live in a manner likely to lead to the gallows. Rope, however, is not the only use to which the fibers can be put; they are extensively employed in clothing, and in the manufacture of paper.

The plant is also cultivated for its seeds, which contain a large quantity of oil, and is therefore used in pharmacy for emulsions, and in the domestic arts because of its drying properties. But the seeds are chiefly used as a favorite food for birds. In fact, some birds consume them to excess, which should lead us to suspect that these seeds, though they cannot intoxicate us, have a narcotic effect on the feathered creatures, making them dream of a happy birdland where there are no gilded cages, and where the men are gunless and the women hatless. The seeds also contain sugar and considerable albumin, making them very nutritious; rabbits eat them readily. They are consumed also by some human beings, but are not as good as the sunflower seeds which Marianka ceaselessly and carelessly crunched, while Olenine looked upon her moving lips with a lover's despair.

The medicinal hemp – the hemp with the potent narcotic principles – is *Cannabis indica.* In this case we have an example of Compensation that would have made Emerson's eyes glisten, for although the fibrous texture of hemp disappears under a southern sun, to make up for the loss there is secreted a resin – *Churrus.* This resin is collected in a most singular manner. During the hot season, according to Dr. O'Shaughnessy, men clothed in leather run violently through the hemp-fields and brush forcibly against the plants. The soft, sticky resin adheres to the garments, and is later scraped off and kneaded into balls. Dr. M'Kinnon informed Dr. O'Shaughnessy that in the province of Nipal the leather attire is dispensed with, and that the natives run naked through the hemp fields, gathering the resin on their bare bodies.

When the larger leaves turn brown and fall to the ground, it is an indication of the approach of maturity. The flowering tops are then cut off, and subjected to a process of rolling and treading by trained human feet. The hemp is placed on a hard floor surrounded by a rail; the natives take hold of a revolving post, march around and around, singing the while, and press the plants in a technical manner. Whether the perspiration which drips from their unshod organs of locomotion works any chemical change in the composition of Cannabis has not yet been determined by E. M. Holmes or E. W. Dixon.

It is not surprising to learn that the dealing in hasheesh is a Government monopoly, and that heavy punishment is meted out to those offenders who buy or sell it without permission. "The importation of it into Egypt is so strongly interdicted," explains the *Dispensatory of the United States*, "that the mere possession of it is a penal offense; we found it, however, readily procurable. It is said to be brought into the country in pigs' bladders, in the Indo-European steamers, and thrown out at night during the passage into the Suez canal, to be picked up by the boats of confederates." This deplorable state of affairs is apt to remind us of our own temperance towns – where there are always some individuals who possess the faculty of obtaining whisky *ad libitum*.

Cannabis sativa is a member of the *Moraceæ* or Mulberry Family, which family was formerly an order of apetalous dicotyledonous trees or shrubs, but is now reduced to a tribe of the *Urticaceæ* or Nettle Family which embraces 110 genera and 1500 species.

Cannabis is an annual herb, and thus endures but one year, because instead of storing away nutritious matter in underground bulbs and tubers like the industrious biennials or perennials, it exultingly expends its new-born energy in the production of beautiful blossoms and the maturation of fruit and seed. "This completed," says Asa Gray, "The exhausted and not at all replenished individual perishes."

Sexually, hemp is diœcious, which means that its staminate and pistillate organs are not on the same plant. When cultivated for its narcotic properties, only the flowering tops of the unfertilized female plants are used, and the male plants are eradicated with great care, as it is claimed that a single one can spoil an entire field – something like a Boccaccion gentleman in a nunnery. The process of weeding out the males is performed by an expert called a poddar, who brings to his work a conscious technical skill, and an unconscious but interesting argument in illustration of what Lester F. Ward has described as the Androcentric World View, for the poddar deliberately reverses the names of the sexes, and designated the useful females as males, and calls the rejected males the females. If we had such impudent poddars in the animal world, no doubt the valuable Jane Addams would be metamorphosed into James, while the unnecessary Mr. Anthony Comstock would be adorned with a feminine appellation.

Cannabis is from 4 to 12 feet in height; its stem is angular, branching, and covered with matted hairs; its leaves are palmate and therefore roughly resemble an open hand; its leaflets are lance-shaped, possessing margins dentated with saw-like teeth; its flowers are yellow and axillary, the male cluster being a raceme and therefore pedicelled, and the female a spike and consequently sessile or stemless; the five male organs or stamens contain pendulous double-celled sacs or anthers; the two female organs or pistils have glandular stigmas, the stigma being the spot where fertilization occurs; the fruit is a gray nut or achene, each containing a single oily seed; the whole plant is covered with a scarcely visible down; the roughness of the leaves and stem is due to the silica, which is a characteristic of the plants of the *Moraceæ*.

Not much need be said of the microscopical characteristics of hemp, for although the powder contains several histological elements, as pollen grains, glands, crystals, resin, fibres, vessels, stone cells, epidermis, parenchyma, – indicating presence of stem, leaf, flower, seed, – its characteristic hairs or trichomes with their cystolith deposits are of sufficient diagnostic value to make it readily recognizable.

Unfortunately, when we come to the chemical constituents of Cannabis, certainty is at an end. As Dorvoult *L'Officine* says, "La composition chimique du cannabis indica est male connue." The conquests of man are peculiar: he lays a cable under the roaring ocean, and he flashes his messages through limitless miles of space; beneath the surface of the earth he rides on an iron horse, and bird-like he sails through the trackless air. But put this common drug before him and he cannot determine its chemical composition. The careful experimenters and the expert assayers are balked.

"I have extracted an alkaloid from hasheesh," says Preobraschensky, "and it is potent." "No, we have found the active constituent," says T. and H. Smith; "it is the resin cannabin." "No," says Personnne, "I have isolated the important ingredient; it is the amber-colored volatile oil, cannabene." "Oh, no," says Frankel, "I have discovered the active principle – it is a phenol aldehyde." "No, indeed," say Wood, Spivey and Easterfield, "it is we who have separated the only active ingredient – it is a red oil, cannabinol." "Oh, not at all," says Hamilton, "not one of these is the active constituent; in fact, the active constituent has not yet been isolated." In such an arena, where the masters dispute, it behooves the amateur to speak with a stammering tongue.

That doubt should prevail on this subject is all the more remarkable when we consider that hemp has been known from a time whereof the mind of man runneth not to the contrary – to use a phrase which seems to delight the lawyers. In the *Odyssey,* a thousand years before the advent of the Christian era, Homer sang of the assuager of grief or Nepenthes, which is believed to have been the hemp-plant. Hemp thus comes ushered into history, held in the beautiful hand of Helen. Hesychius narrates that the Thracian women made sheets of hemp. Pliny says hemp was known to the Romans, who manufactured cordage from it. The Father of History relates that the Scythians threw the seeds of hemp on red-hot stones, and bathed themselves in the vapor, crying with exultation. Moschion records that the ship *Syracusia*, built for Hiero – kinsman of

Archimedes – was rigged with hempen ropes. In the most ancient of all Hindu medical works, *Susruta*, hemp is recommended for catarrh. The Pandit Moodoosudun Gooptu found in the *Rajni-guntu* a clear account of hemp. A Sanscrit work on Materia Medica, *Rajbulubha*, alludes to the use of hemp in gonorrhea. According to Kamalakantha Vidyalanka, hemp was early forbidden to pious Brahmins. The old Arabic and Persian writers made numerous references to cannabis, and declared its narcotic properties were discovered by Haider. Haider was a rigid monk who built a monastery on the mountains between Nishabor and Ramah. For ten years he never left his hermitage, never indulged in even a fleeting moment's pleasure. One burning summer's day when the fiery sun glared angrily upon Mother Earth as if he wished to wither up her breasts, Haider stepped out from his cloister and walked alone to the fields. All around him lay the vegetation weary and without life, but one plant danced in the heat with joy. Haider plucked it, partook of it, and returned to the convent a happier man. The monks who saw him immediately noticed the change in their chief. He encouraged conversation, and acted boisterously. He then led his companions to the fields, and the holy men partook of the hasheesh, and were transformed from austere ascetics into jolly good fellows. At the death of Haider, in conformity with his desire, his disciples planted the hemp in an arbor around his tomb.

In that portion of the Chinese herbal, *Rh-ya*, which was written 500 B.C., the seed and flower-bearing kinds of hemp are noticed. In the first century, Dioscorides – the most renowned of the ancient writers on the Materia Medica – recommended the seeds in the form of a cataplasm to soothe inflammation. In the second century, Galen wrote that it was customary to give hemp to guests at banquets to promote hilarity and happiness. At the beginning of the third century, the physician Hoa–Thoa used hemp as an anesthetic in surgical operations. In the thirteenth century, garments of hemp became common throughout Southern Europe, and it may well be that Beatrice herself wore it when Dante first saw the maiden in her father's house.

There is a remarkable episode in the history of hasheesh, indicating how the character of a people may be affected by the surrounding vegetation. Mohammediannism, like all other theologies, has been rent by schisms, and the question as to who was the legitimate successor of the Prophet split this Oriental faith into two great sects – the Sunnis and the Shiahs. The latter were the heretics, as they considered Mohammed's son-in-law the true imam. The Shiahs themselves were further subdivided into several parties, the Ismaelites being the most important. The Ismaelites were especially powerful in Persia, and later – through the instrumentality of an escaped prisoner who seized the throne – gained a firm foothold in Egypt. A grand lodge was formed in the city of Cairo – on the banks of the river whose ancient waters heard the hammering at the quarries for the rearing of the Great Pyramid. Many rules were now made by the Ismaelites, and the petty race of perishable men was must flustered, while the immortal Nile flowed indifferently from its equatorial cradle, refreshing the crimson water-lillies, bathing the reeds that lined its shore, and wetting the sands where the thoughtful Sphinx opens not its lips.

In the course of time this lodge was visited by the clever Ismaelite, Hassan Ben Sabbah – a boyhood friend of Omar Khayyám – who was received with acclamation. Hassan soon received enough honors to excite jealousy, and while plotting for more power was defeated and forced to disappear from Egypt, but, after traveling awhile, he settled near Kuhistan. He gathered around him a considerable number of followers, and by strategy, in 1090, captured the powerful Persian fortress of Alamut. Hassan now introduced a new feature into his society – the employment of secret murder against all enemies. It was the Sheikh of this organization who loomed large in medieval folk-lore as the Old Man of the Mountains. Many young men became disciples, and willingly performed the bloody work. These youths were known as the Fedais or Devoted Ones. When a Devoted One was selected to commit the murder, he was first stupified with hasheesh, and while in this state was brought into the magnificent gardens of the sheikh. All the sensual and stimulating pleasures of the erotic orient surrounded the excited youth and, exalted by the delicious hypnotic he had taken, the hot-blooded fanatic felt that the gates of heaven were already ajar, and heard them swing open on their golden hinges. When the effect of the drug disappeared and the Devoted One was reduced to his normal condition, he was informed that through the generosity of his superior he had been permitted to foretaste the delights of Paradise. The Devoted One believed this readily enough – disciples are always credulous – and therefore was eager to die or to kill at a word from his master. From these hasheesh-eaters, the Arabian name of which is *hashshashin*, was derived the term "assassin." It is not known at what date the epithet was first applied to other secret slayers. The Assassins soon became a terrible scourge, and the very sands of the desert almost learned to tremble before them. Many an unprepared breast felt their daggers, and may a surprised stomach tried in vain to vomit up their poisons. Prince and calif they struck down, and more than one haughty chief paid tribute to the Old Man of the Mountains. During the invasion of Palestine by the Crusaders, the Syrian branch of the Assassins reached its bloody zenith, and who shall say how many high-born damsels wept for knightly shields that lay low in the dust of Lebanon? The power of the Assassins was destroyed in Persia about the middle of the thirteenth century, and some years later the Mameluke sultan of Egypt exterminated them in Syria. But just as there are still some Innsbruck Jesuits who pray for the revival of the Spanish Inquisition, so some remnants of the Assassins yet linger between the Tigris river and the mount of Taurus – but what of that? The Old Man of the Mountains now sleeps in Death's Valley, and not all the hasheesh from Bengal could exalt him.

Towards the end of the eighteenth century, when Napoleon invaded Egypt – and grew philosophic as he met the gaze of the prehistoric pyramids – hasheesh was brought prominently to the notice of Europeans by the accounts of DeSacy and Rouger. By this time its narcotic properties must have been known to the Occidentals, for as far back as 1690 Berlu in his *Treasury of Drugs* described it as "of an infatuating quality and pernicious use." Nevertheless, its introduction into the Pharmacopeias of Europe and the United States is due mainly to the elaborate experimentation carried on during 1839 and several succeeding years by the talented Dr. William B. O'Shaughnessy, Professor of Chemistry in the Medical College of Calcutta.

This brings us to the physiological action of Cannabis. It primarily stimulates the brain, has a mydriatic effect upon the pupil, slightly accelerates the pulse, sometimes quickens and sometimes retards breathing, produces a ravenous appetite, increases the amount of urine, and augments the contractions of the uterus. In other words, it has an effect on the nervous, respiratory, circulatory, digestive, excretory and genito-urinary systems.

As a therapeutic agent hasheesh has its eulogizers, though like many other drugs it has been replaced by later remedies in various disorders for which it was formerly used. Old drugs, like old folks, must give way to the new, and even the therapeutic master-builders must beware when the young generation of healing-agents knocks on the door of health.

In medicinal doses Cannabis is used as an aphrodisiac, for neuralgia, to quiet maniacs, for the cure of chronic alcoholism and morphine and chloral habits, for mental depression, hysteria, softening of the brain, nervous vomiting, for distressing cough, for St. Vitus' dance, and for the falling sickness so successfully simulated by Kipling's Sleary – epileptic fits of a most appalling kind. It is used in spasm of the bladder, in migrane, and when the dreaded Bacillus tetanus makes the muscles rigid. It is a uterine tonic, and a remedy in the headaches and hemorrhages occurring at the final cessation of the menses. It has been pressed into the service of the diseases that mankind has named in honor of Venus. According to Osler, Cannabis is sometimes useful in locomotor ataxia. Christison reports a case in which Cannabis entirely cured the intense itching of eczema, while the patient was enjoying the delightful slumber which the hemp induced. It is much employed as a hypnotic in those cases where opium because of long-continued use has lost its efficiency. As a specific in hydrophobia it is sometimes marvelous, for Dr. J. W. Palmer writes that he himself has seen a sepoy, an hour before furiously hydrophobic, under the influence of cannabis drinking water freely and pleasantly washing his face and hands! its function in this unspeakable affliction should be investigated carefully, for it will be a gala day for mankind when it can cease to fear Montaigne's terrible line: "The saliva of a wretched dog touching the hand of Socrates, might disturb and destroy his intellect."

The official definition of *Cannabis indica* as given by the Eighth Decennial Revision of our *Pharmacopeia* is as follows: "The dried flowering tops of the pistillate plants of *Cannabis sativa* Linné (Fam. *Moraceæ*), grown in the East Indies and gathered while the fruits are yet undeveloped, and carrying the whole of their natural resin." Three preparations of the drug are official: an Extract, a Fluid extract, and a Tincture.

In the last (third) edition of the *National Formulary,* hemp enters into four galenicals: in chloral and bromine compound which is used as a sedative and hypnotic, in chloroform Anodyne which is used in diarrhea and cholera, in Brown-Sequard's anti-neuralgic pills, and in corn collodion. Hemp is a constituent in the majority of corn remedies. Not many drugs are used for both the brain and the feed, but with Cannabis we have this anomaly: a man may see visions by swallowing his corn-cure.

Out of the enormous number of prescriptions in which hasheesh enters as an ingredient, only half-a-dozen can be here represented. In Hager's *Pharmaceustische Praxis* occurs this prescription for gonorrhea:

℞

Kali nitrici
Natri nitrici ana 5,0
Extracti Hyoscyami 0,5
Aquæ Amygdalarum amararum 10,0
Emulsionis Cannabis fructus 200,0

For dysmenorrhea the *Journal de Médecine de Paris* recommends the following suppositories, with the directions that one be introduced every evening, commencing with the fifth day before the menses:

℞

Ex. cannab. indicæ   . . . gr. ¼
Ex. belladonnæ   . . . gr. ¼
Ol. theobrom   . . . q. s. – M.

For phthisis, when accompanied by insomnia and nervous dyspepsia, Dr. S. G. Bonney prescribes:

℞

Strychnin. sulph.   . . . gr. 2/3
Extracti opii   . . . gr. j

Extracti cannabis indicæ.. . . gr. j ss
Salolis   . . . gr. c.
Aloini   . . . gr. ss. – M.
Pone in capsulas No. xx

Dr. Rankin fights dyspepsia with the following formula, one capsule being given after meals:

R

Zinci valeratis   . . . ʒj
Acidi carbolici   . . . gr. xl
Acidi arsenosi   . . . gr. ss
Extracti cannabis indicæ . . . gr. v. – M.
Pone in capsulas No. xx.

When a patient of Van Harlingen is attacked with *ichthyosis hystriæ*, the disagreeable skin-disease finds itself daily painted with this preparation:

R

Acid. salicylici   . . . ʒss
Ex. cannabis ind.   . . . gr. x
Collodii   . . . fℨj – M

Dr. Da Costa endeavors to relieve impotence by giving his patients, morning and evening, this pill:

R

Ex. cannabis indicæ   . .
Ex. nucis vomicæ   . . . aa gr. xv
Ex. ergotae aquosi   . . . ʒj. – M.
Et. ft. pil. No. xxx

The results of the prolonged use of large doses of Cannabis are thus epitomized by Alfred Stillé: "The habitual use of this drug entails consequences no less mischievous than are produced by alcohol and opium; the face becomes bloated, the eyes injected, the limbs weak and tremulous, the mind sinks into a state of imbecility, and death by marasmus is the ultimate penalty paid for the over-strained pleasure it imparts."

Poisoning by hasheesh is treated by the administration of emetics (what poison isn't), lemon-juice, tannin, coffee, ammonia, strychnine, atropine, spirit of nitrous ether. Electricity and artificial respiration are often useful.

A strange thing about hasheesh is that an overdose has never produced death in man or the lower animals. Not one authentic case is on record in which Cannabis or any of its preparations destroyed life. We thus have a poison which lacks a maximum and a fatal dose. Indeed, if we desire to be finical, we can claim that according to what is now considered the best definition of a poison, Cannabis is no poison at all, for the aforesaid best definition defines a poison as "any substance which is capable of causing death, otherwise than mechanically, when introduced into the body or applied to it" – and Cannabis does not seem capable of causing death by chemical or physiological action.

"Hemp," says Professor Horatio C. Wood, "is not a dangerous drug; even the largest doses of its active preparations, although causing most alarming symptoms, do not compromise life."

"We have never been able," testify Drs. Houghton and Hamilton, "to give an animal a sufficient quantity of the drug to produce death. When study of the drug was first commenced, careful search on the literature of the subject was made to determine its toxicity. Not a single case of fatal poisoning have we been able to find reported, although often alarming symptoms may occur. A dog weighing about 25 pounds received an injection of 2 ounces of the U. S. P. fluidextract in the jugular vein, with the expectation that it would certainly be sufficient to kill the animal. To our surprise the animal after being unconscious for about a day and a half, recovered completely. Another dog received about 7 grams of the solid extract with the same result."

That herbivorous animals are even less affected by it I know from my own simple experiments. I gave a rabbit a drachm and a half of the fluidextract of Cannabis. No sooner did I release the animal than it begin to nibble a commonplace vegetable, indifferent to the circumstance that it had been baptised with the most precious opiate of the orient. For four hours I watched this member of the genus *Lepus*, but no physical effects could be observed, while the mild expression of its gentle eyes induced me to conclude that all mental manifestations were lacking to such a degree that the bunny still worshipped the rather material trinity of crackers, carrots and cabbages. This rabbit was sold to an experienced dealer, and sometime later while passing the store, I learned it had become the sire of a goodly progeny, but what I really would like to learn is this: will those little innocent rabbits – with their asinine ears and angelic eyes – ever know of their father's enforced hasheesh debauch?

Few creatures have so slight a hold on life as the pretty guinea-pig – which does not come from Guinea and is not a pig. A blow of the hand, a bit of moisture, a breath of cold, and their squealing is done. But they do not mind Cannabis. I chose a fine fellow, anesthetized his glossy back with ethyl chloride, and then by means of a hypodermic syringe injected 100 minims of the powerful fluidextract into his circulation. There were no results. After the elapse of some hours the generous cavy so far forgot the incident as to pull some sweet-pea pods from my hand.

Dr. O'Shaughnessy says that all his experiments "tended to demonstrate that, while carnivorous animals and fish, dogs, cats, swine, vultures, crows, and adjutants invariably and speedily exhibited the intoxicating influence of the drug, the graminivorous, such as the horse, deer, monkey, goat, sheep, and cow, experienced but trivial effects from any dose we administered." Lieutaud and Mabillat say the same.

Up to this period we have considered hasheesh from the historic, botanic, microscopic, chemic, physiologic, therapeutic and pharmacologic viewpoints: what then remains? Why, friends, the best is yet to be, the last for which the first was made – as Browning would say.

Why has everyone heard of opium? Because of its somnifacient and myotic properties? No, but because sixty million pounds are consumed by people for the purpose of pleasure. It is the same with hasheesh. All heathens use it to increase their joys: Moors, Mohammedans, Malays, Burmese, Siamese, Hindoos, Hottentots, Australian Bushmen and Brazilian Indians – three hundred millions of them. The grateful Orientals have endowed their hasheesh with such epithets as exciter of desire, increaser of pleasure, cementer of friendship, leaf of delusion, the laughter-mover, causer of the reeling gait. "It is real happiness," says Monsieur Moreau, and Herbert Spencer quotes the sentence in his *Principles of Psychology,* – "It is real happiness which hasheesh causes."

It is unreasonable to suppose that a powerful narcotic like Cannabis will produce uniform results in all instances, when it is notorious that even coffee affects different people in different ways; one lady drinks tea to keep her awake at night, and her neighbor drinks it to put her asleep; a Havana cigar irritates Brown and tranquilizes Jones; a glass of grog causes one man to beat his children, and induces another to give away his coat to strangers. The constitutional peculiarity of the subject must always be taken into consideration: some folks are so absurd as to become afflicted with nettle-rash after partaking of delicious strawberries; others are poisoned by an egg; some become ill in the presence of the violet, and others faint when they smell the lily; Tissot mentions a person who vomited if he took a grain of sugar; Louis XIV had grand manners, but he preferred the odor of cat's urine to that of the red rose. "Jack Sprat could eat no fat, his wife could eat no lean." Idiosyncrasy may not be the star performer, but it certainly plays an important rôle in the therapeutic drama.

No drug in the entire Materia Medica is capable of producing such a diversity of effects as Cannabis indica. "Of the action of hasheesh," writes Professor Stillé, "many and various descriptions have been given which differ so widely among themselves that they would scarcely be supposed to apply to the same agent, had we not every day a no less remarkable instance of the same kind before us in the case of alcohol. As the latter enlivens or saddens, excites or depresses, fills with tenderness, or urges to brutality, imparts vigor and activity, or nauseates and weakens, so does the former give rise to even a still greater variety of phenomena, according to the natural disposition of the person, and his existing state of mind, the quantity of the drug, and the combinations in which it is taken."

And not only is there a contrariety and dissimilarity of action, but sometimes there is no action at all. Cannabis is certainly the coquette of drugdom. Take agaric, and it will stop your perspiration – take jaborandi, and it will sweat you half to death; take creosote, and it will prevent emesis – take ipecac, and it will vomit you till your very guts cry out for mercy; take eserine, and your pupils will contract – take atropine, and they will dilate; veratrine will make you sneeze, the dust of sanguinaria will give you a bloody nose, aloes will act on your lower bowel, podophyllum will work on the upper, squill will make you pass water by the quart, an injection of strychnine will stimulate you, a dose of morphine will put you in the arms of Morpheus, – but take Cannabis, and who can predict the result? It may do wondrous things to you, and it may let you strictly alone.

To a worker on the Associated Press named I. M. Norr, I gave 30 minims of the fluidextract. There were no results. To a law student named Aaron Wolman, I gave 40 minims. There was no more effect than if he had taken 40 drops of water. It must be added, however, that these experimenters, instead of putting themselves in a receptive state, had determined beforehand to fight the influence of the drug. On the evening of May 18, 1910, I gave 25 minims to Dr. Anna Mercy, and although she threw herself at the shrine of science in a way that must have astonished the sober old altar of experiment, there were no results worth mentioning, except that while in the evening she looked respectable, in the morning she looked disreputable.

Had all my experiments turned out thus, this essay would never have been written. But I have had results fully as interesting as those achieved by O'Shaughnessy, Moreau, Mabillat, Reidel, Schroff, Wood, Bell, Christison, Aubert, and many others, including our gifted traveler-poet Bayard Taylor.

My brother Frederic Robinson took 25 minims in the presence of some ladies whom he had invited to witness the fun. An hour passed without results. A second hour followed, but – to use the slang of the street – there was nothing doing. The third hour promised to be equally fruitless, and as it was already late in the evening, the ladies said good-by. No sooner did they leave the room, than I heard the hasheesh-laugh. The hemp was doing its work. In a shrill voice my brother was exclaiming, "What foo-oolish people, what foo-oo-ool-ish people to leave just when the show is beginning." The ladies came back. And it was a show. Frederic made Socialistic speeches, and argued warmly for the cause of Woman Suffrage. He grew most affectionate and insisted on holding a lady's hand. His face was flushed, his eyes were half closed, his abdomen seemed uneasy, but his spirit was happy. He sang, he rhymed, he declaimed, he whistled, he mimicked, he acted. He pleaded so passionately for the rights of Humanity that it seemed he was using up the resources of his system. But he was tireless. With both hands he gesticulated, and would brook no interruption.

Peculiar ideas suggested themselves. For instance, he said something was "sheer nonsense," and then reasoned as follows: "Since shears are the same as scissors, instead of sheer nonsense I can say scissors nonsense." He also said, "I will give you a kick in the tickle" – and was much amused by the expression.

At all times he recognized those about him, and remained conscious of his surroundings. When the approach of dawn forced the ladies to depart, Frederic made a somewhat unsavory joke, and immediately exclaimed triumphantly, "I wouldn't have said that if the ladies were here for a million dollars." Someone yawned deeply, and being displeased by the unexpected appearance of a gaping orifice, Frederic melodramatically gave utterance to this Gorky-like phrase: "From the depths of dirtiness and despair there rose a sickly odorous yawn" – and instantly he remarked that the first portion of this sentence was alliterative! Is it not strange that such consciousness and such intoxication can exist in the same brain simultaneously?

The next day he remembered all that occurred, was in excellent spirits, laughed much and easily, and felt himself above the petty things of this world.

On May 13, 1910, this world was excited over the visit of Halley's comet. It is pleasant to remember that the celestial guest attracted as much attention as a political campaign or a game of baseball. On the evening of this day, at 10 o'clock, I gave 45 minims to a court stenographer named Henry D. Demuth. At 11:30 the effects of the drug became apparent, and Mr. Demuth lost consciousness of his surroundings to such an extent that he imagined himself an inhabitant of Sir Edmund Halley's nebulous planet. He despised the earth and the dwellers thereon; he called it a miserable little flea-bite, and claimed its place in the cosmos was no more important than a flea–jump. With a scornful finger he pointed below, and said in a voice of contempt, "That little joke down there, called the earth."

"Victor," he said, "you're a fine fellow, you're the smartest man in Harlem, you've got the god in you, but the best thoughts you write are low compared to the things we think up here." A little later he condescended to take me up with him, and said, "Victor, we're up in the realm now, and we'll make money when we get down on that damned measly earth again; they respect Demuth on earth."

He imitated how Magistrate Butts calls a prisoner to the bar. "Butts," he explained, "is the best of them. Butts – Butts – cigarette-butts." If this irreverent line should ever fall beneath the dignified eyes of His Honor, instead of fining his devoted stenographer for contempt of court, may he bear in his learned mind the fact that under the influence of narcotics men are mentally irresponsible.

By this time Mr. Demuth's vanity was enormous "God, Mark Twain and I are chums," he remarked casually. "God is wise, and I am wise. And to think that people *dictate* to me!"

He imagined he had material for a great book. "I'm giving you the thoughts; slap them down, we'll make a fortune and go whacks. We'll make a million. I'll get half and Vic will get half. With half a million we'll take it easy for a while on this damned measly earth. We'll live till a hundred and two, and then we'll skedaddle didoo. At one hundred and two it will be said of Henry Disque Demuth that he shuffled off this mortal coil. We'll skip into the great idea – hooray! hooray! Take down everything that is signifi*cant* – with an accent on the cant – Immanuel Kant was a wise man, and I'm a wise man; I am wise, because I'm wise."

It is to be regretted that in spite of all the gabble concerning the volume that was to make both of us rich, not even one line was dictated by the inspired author. In fact he got no further than the title, and it must be admitted that of all titles in the world, this is the least catchy. It is as follows: "Wise is God; God is Wise."

Later came a variation in the form of a hissing sound which was meant to be an imitation of the whizzing of Halley's comet; there was a wild swinging of the sheets as a welcome to the President; a definition of religion as the greatest joke ever perpetrated; some hasheesh-laughter; and the utterance of this original epigram: Shakespeare, seltzer-beer, be cheerful.

A little later all variations ceased, for the subject became a monomaniac, or at any rate, a fanatic. He became thoroughly imbued with the great idea that the right attitude to preserve towards life is to take all things on earth as a joke. Hundreds and hundreds and hundreds of times he repeated: "The idea of the great idea, the idea of the great idea, the idea of the great idea." No question could steer him out of this track. "Who's up on the comet? Any pretty girls there?" asked Frederic. "The great idea is up there," was the answer.

"Where would you fall if you fell off the comet!"

"I'd fall into the great idea."

"What do you do when you want to eat and have no money?"

"You have to get the idea."

"When will you get married?"

"When I get the idea."

Midnight came, and he was still talking about his great idea. At one o'clock I felt bored. "If you don't talk about anything else except the idea, we'll have to quit," I said.

"Yes," he replied, "we'll all quit, we'll all be wrapped up in the great idea." He took out his handkerchief to blow his nose, remarking, "The idea of my nose." I approached him. "Don't interfere," he cried, "I'm off with the great idea."

I began to descend the stairs. When halfway down I stopped to listen. He was still a monomaniac. Had he substituted the word thought or theory or conception or notion or belief or opinion or supposition or hypothesis or syllogism or tentative conjecture, I would have returned. But as I still heard only the idea of the great idea, I went to bed.

In the morning his countenance was ashen, which formed a marked contrast to its extreme redness the evening before. He should have slept longer, but I thought of the duties to be performed for Judge Butts, and determined to arouse him, although I knew my touch would cast him down from the glorious Halley's comet to the measly little flea-bite of an earth, besides jarring the idea of the great idea.

So I shook him, but instead of manifesting anger, he smiled and extended his hand cordially, as if he had not seen me for a long time. The effects of the drug had not entirely disappeared, and his friends at work thought him drunk, and asked with whom he had been out all night. Mr. Demuth was in first-class spirits, he bubbled over with idealism, and felt a contempt for all commercial transactions. He was the American Bernard Shaw, and looked upon the universe as a joke of the gods. While adding some figures of considerable importance – as salaries depended upon the results – a superintendent passed. Mr. Demuth pointed to the column that needed balancing, and asked, "This is all a joke, isn't it!" Not appreciating the etiology of the query, the superintendent nodded and passed on.

One midnight, while preparing to retire, it occurred to Courtenay Lemon that this was a good time for him to try hasheesh. As I did not discourage him in the slightest degree, 30 minims were forthwith swallowed, with the result that the Socialist dramatic critic spent an unusual night. It must be remarked that over the bed on which he lay hangs a portrait of Ralph Waldo Emerson. For an hour and a quarter we discussed various topics of mutual interest, such as decadent poetry, and Marx's influence on the revolutionary youth of Russia. The conversation was cut short by the hasheesh-laugh.

It had begun: the flood of laughter was loose, the deluge of mirth poured forth, the cascard of cachinnation rushed on till it swelled into a torrent of humor while the waves of snickering and tittering mingled with the freshets of hilarity and jollity till the whole poured into a marvelous Niagara of merriment. What a pity the audience was so small! What a shame the old humorists could not be present! How the belly of Aristophanes would have thundered a loud *papapappax*, how Scarron would have grinned, how Sydney Smith would have enjoyed it, how Tom Moore would have held his aching sides, how Rabelais would have raised the rafters with his loud ho-ho-hos! But as these gentlemen were unavoidably detained elsewhere, I must testify that it was the funniest show on earth, – so here's to you, Courtenay Lemon, you Leyden jar of laughter, charged to the limit.

Never having been a disciple of good old Isaac Pitman, I could not record all that was said, but here are my notes: "I feel a satisfaction," he says, "in seeing Emerson's picture, as I always felt like laughing at him." Rolls on the bed and laughs uncontrollably. "It makes my face tired," he explains. In reply to my question, he answers that he enjoys laughing. Begins to expound something but is stopped by a laughing fit. Says he would like to have his photo taken now, and then laughs immoderately. Says it doesn't seem so much like laughing as like letting wind out of a bag. Says it is worth while staying up to see such a show. Giggles terrifically. Says "Open the window, as I am using up all the air." Laughs loud and long. Strangely enough his laughter begins to sound exactly like a negro's, as represented on the stage. He recognizes this and says: "I'se laughin' now jes' like a niggah." He is extraordinarily comical. From top to bottom his body is shaking with laughter. He twirls his arms, kicks his feet, and for the first time I understand what Milton meant when he wrote "the light fantastic toe."

"I feel as if any way I put my leg I have to keep it. If I stuck it in the air and kept it there – wouldn't that be funny?" Loud laughing. Imitates the music of a military band. His eyes glisten with pleasure, his whole countenance is beaming, and he seems infinitely delighted with himself. "Foreward march!" he exclaims. He plays a fife and beats a drum: Boom! Boom! Boom! Says sternly, "I don't want this band to play any patriotic air, not even in my sleep."

"Ladies and gentlemen, I tell you a story. You think I'm a damn fool, don't you?" Laughter. "This reminds me of a story." Laughter. "O what a damn fool am I!" Laughter. "I'm going to tell that story," he says determinedly. Makes several attempts, but it is a difficult feat, on account of the frequent outbursts of laughter, and because it is next to impossible for him to concentrate his thoughts. At last he gets this out: "A man said he hadn't laughed so much since his mother-in-law died. Oh, how funny!"

"Mr. Courtenay Lemon: Imitation of laughter. Pretty good, eh?" Makes a speech, imitates the gestures, and bows as politely as it is possible for one who is stretched out in bed.

"This would be a good dope to try on a fellow who is accused of having no sense of humor. Oh, I'm getting funnier every minute."

"Emerson, O you, you were a kid once too, weren't you? I don't believe you ever were. If I had a rotten egg I'd throw it at you."

"There's a blue phosphorescent light in your face –"

"I'd rather laugh than vomit any day." Strikes the bowl which was placed near him in case the Cannabis produced emesis. "But I'm not a dog and I'll not return to my vomit. That dog was a damn fool. There are a lot of things in the Bible that are damn fool things."

"I've been doing all sorts of laughter. Couldn't you have a system of prosody, and divide it off into feet like poetry, and have a Laughing Poet whose contributions would be accepted by the comic papers?" Whistles and sings and drums rhythmically with his finger-tips on the bowl.

When I confirm a statement of his by answering "Yes," he says, "Don't be butting in, Victor, this is my show." Points his finger at me and laughs. Sensations must be very acute, for while clearing my throat to say something, but before uttering anything, he hears me and exclaims: "There you go, butting in again. But don't be afraid, I'm not getting pugnacious; it all ends in laughter." But for a moment does become quarrelsome.

"I had a good thought, but I don't know what's best: to stick to the thought or stick to the laughter?"

"If Chauncey Depew should be wrecked in the New York Central, wouldn't that be funny? Would it be poetic justice? No, it would be the justice of laughter. Oh, it would be the laughter of the gods!" He raises himself and swings his arm dramatically. Laughter leaps from his insides as if it were a geyser spouting up, and rushes from his lips as if it were a cataract bounding down a boulder.

He theorizes about egoism and Max Stirner, but I can not jot down the reflection in its entirety.

He says I have no sense of humor to sit there taking notes, instead of joining him in laughing.

"Of course you understand why I am laughing. But your old cook – if she hears me, she'll send for the police."

"It's too bad that when I'm having such a good time, I should be troubled by a dry taste in the mouth. It's another evidence that the world was created by a damn fool or a lunatic. There is always some little thing that interferes."

Talks sensibly awhile, and then says impatiently: "I want to stop all this talking, and get to laughing again. I'm not complaining about the effects from hasheesh, because I consider it worth everything."

"Oh, tell me, pretty maiden, why can't a little canary bird whistle a symphony, for instance, Tchaikovsky's *Le Pathetique*?" Whistles, waves his hand fantastically. "As damn little as I know about music, not having been gifted by nature in that direction" – twists his arms in a grotesque manner – "I'm able to get a bunch out of Tchaikovsky. I don't mean comrade Tchaikovsky, the revolutionist in Russia, I mean Peter Ilich Tchaikovsky. The itch of that Ilich – it seems like a personal ailment, it sounds insulting."

Throws a piece of paper at me, but says, "Don't be afraid, I'll break no bones."

I ask him to tell the time. He gazes intently at the clock, and says, "I want to get it exactly on the fraction of a second. But it changes so quickly, I can't." Gives it up in disgust.

Claims a heavy feeling is creeping over him, and wonders if it is due to increased blood pressure. "But what am I beginning to talk serious for? I could keep on laughing for a couple of weeks, except that I don't want to keep you up."

"If Spencer had been more of a sport and had taken some of this stuff, he would have had material for his essay, *The Physiology of Laughter.*" To see a man drugged with hasheesh quoting the profoundest of synthetic philosophers is too much for my gravity, and for a moment my scream of laughter eclipses even his.

"Ah, I'm beginning to get light again. It's much nicer to be light and delicate. To be a filmy butterfly, and float in fancy," – his face assumes an expression of poetic beauty, and he speculates whether man should live a life of beauty or of duty.

"Oh, I'm willing to laugh…" Throws off the blankets and cries. "Throw off the bonds of all existence!"

I ask him what day it is. "I hope," says he, with a melodramatic wave of the hand, "I will express the modest hope, that in accordance to my wishes, and in conformity to my desires, it is Sunday night! Sunday night! Sunday night!"

Sits up, looks at me rougishly and laughs.

"I feel a metalliferous touch within me. I'd rather have a cramp in my leg than in my brain. Some people would call this a brain-cramp, wouldn't they?" Laughs, kicks up his legs.

"If you got erotic while laughing, wouldn't it be blasphemy? Worse than laughing in church."

"Have no illusions of death yet. I am still in a position to laugh death in the face, to laugh…" – and he proves it. He claps his hands together merrily.

Has a lucid moment, looks at the clock, and says simply and correctly, "10 to 3."

Imitates a Frenchman most admirably, accent, gestures, etc.

The door opens, and my father – who has found it impossible to sleep with a roaring volcano in the house – enters. I ask Mr. Lemon to tell my father about Chauncey Depew and the Grand Central. Mr. Lemon is highly pleased, and repeats the story with intense zest. He enlarges it, and claims Depew has got Elbert Hubbard beat as a hypocrite. He says all who believe Depew deserves to be killed should signify it by saying Aye, and then he himself, as if he were a whole assembly, shouts out, Aye! Aye! Aye! "The Ayes have it," he announces with the air of a man who has just won an important victory. My father and I laugh heartily. There is no limit to Mr. Lemon's happiness. "That's right," he says, "it's good, take it down, old man."

He cannot bear a moment's abstinence from laughter. "Cast aside all irrelevant hypotheses, and get to the laughing. I proclaim the supremacy of the laugh, laughter inextinguishable, laughter eternal, the divine laughter of the gods."

My father leaves the room. "Everything has a comic element if you look at it right. It seemed to me that your father went down into the cellar because he couldn't sleep on account of my damn foolishness." He wallows in amusement, but at the same time expresses sincere regret that he is preventing my father and me from sleeping, and says next time he will take hasheesh in the daytime.

My father re-enters, and desires to feel his pulse. At first Mr. Lemon objects vehemently to being touched, but then smiles the sweetest of smiles, and with the demeanor of a martyred Bruno marching to the stake, stretches forth his hand, saying, "In the interests of science I am willing." But after a few seconds Mr. Lemon pulls his hand impatiently away, and exclaims angrily, "You've been holding it a half an hour." His pulse is about 100.

"Come on in, the hasheesh is fine! You laugh and laugh and laugh and laugh like an imbecile. Who can laugh in more ways than me? Not any fellow that I can see."

Begins to philosophize about savages, but loses the threat of his thoughts. I remind him what he was talking about; he thinks a moment, taps his forehead significantly, and says, "There was a laugh there before, and now I've lost it."

"Every tick of the clock is another instant that you're wasting time over this damn foolishness."

"Laughter is indisputable and for its own sake. I proclaim the laugh for the laugh's sake." The English tongue is insufficient for him; he coins words of his own: "Laughfinity!" he shouts. "Laughinosity!" he screams. "The whole world is a blooming joke."

"Which is best," he asks innocently, "the laughing Goddess, or the Goddess of Laughter?" "The Laughing Goddess," answers my father. Exultation shines through the dilated pupils fo the questioner, as he responds, "I knew I would catch you. The Laughing Goddess reminds you by the association of ideas of the laughing hyena, and then instead of being the goddess presiding over the divine function of laughter, she becomes a laughing stock."

I ask him something about figures. "Figures," he answers, "are intellectually beneath me. In short, I would never be a great mathematician. Yet I appreciate the metaphysics of mathematics. I adore, I prostrate myself before mathematics as long as there are no figures in it." Hearing our laughter, he explains, "Yet this isn't so foolish as it seems. Up to a certain point in geometry there are no figures."

"I would have talked more sensibly if Emerson had not been there." Bangs his legs against the edge of the bed; my father asks him if he hurt himself. "Not on a material plane; it was a psychic jar of which you cannot conceive."

Speaks in a declamatory tone: "I am all the time on the border-line between Science and Folly. Which god shall ye follow, young man?"

My father tells him he can stop laughing if he wishes. "No, sir," comes the emphatic response, "not if you lived in my world. It is a categorical imperative in the world of hasheesh: Thou shalt laugh."

It is already four o'clock in the morning. I am loath to leave this frolicsome dynamo of blithesomeness, this continuous current of good cheer, this generator of joyousness, but there is a hard day's work before me and I need a little sleep, so with a last look at his Mirthful Majesty, I leave him alone in his glory and his giggles.

Four hours later I peep in. The intellectual merry-andrew who criticizes the Concord Transcendentalist and juggles philosophic conceptions even under the effects of dope, is motionless. Lassitude has usurped the throne of laughter.

I cannot tell what effect the reading of this case will produce on others, but in me it awakens such risibility that I hope never to think of it on an occasion when silence or solemnity is enjoined; for if I do, there is danger of my being ejected as unceremoniously as was

Washington Irving on the day he laughed at *The Art of Book Making*, in the grave sanctuary of the British Museum.

There yet remains my own case. On March 4, 1910, I came home, feeling very tired. I found that some Cannabis indica which I had expected had arrived. After supper, while finishing up an article, I began to debate with myself whether I should join the hasheesh-eaters that night. The argument ended in my taking 20 minims at 9 o'clock. I was alone in the room, and no one was aware that I had yielded to temptation. An hour later I wrote in my memoranda book: Absolutely no effect. At 10:30, I completed my article, and entered this note: No effect at all from the hemp. By this time I was exhausted, and being convinced that the hasheesh would not act, I went to bed in disappointment. I fell asleep immediately.

I hear music. There is something strange about this music. I have not heard such music before. The anthem is far away, but in its very faintness there is a lure. In the soft surge and swell of the minor notes there breathes a harmony that ravishes the sense of sound. A resonant organ, with a stop of sapphire and a diapason of opal, diffuses endless octaves from star to star. All the moonbeams form strings to vibrate the perfect pitch, and this entrancing unison is poured into my enchanted ears. Under such a spell, who can remain in bed? The magic of that melody bewitches my soul. I begin to rise horizontally from my couch. No walls impede my progress, and I float into the outside air. Sweeter and sweeter grows the music, it bears me higher and higher, and I float in tune with the infinite – under the turquoise heavens where globules of mercury are glittering.

I become an unhindered wanderer through unending space. No air-ship can go here, I say. I am astonished at the vastness of infinity. I always knew it was large, I argue, but I never dreamed it was as huge as this. I desire to know how fast I am floating through the air, and I calculate that it must be about a billion miles a second.

I am transported to wonderland. I walk in streets where gold is dirt, and I have no desire to gather it. I wonder whether it is worth while to explore the canals of Mars, or rock myself on the rings of Saturn, but before I can decide, a thousand other fancies enter my excited brain.

I wish to see if I can concentrate my mind sufficiently to recite something, and I succeed in correctly quoting this stanza from a favorite poem which I am perpetually re-reading:

> "Come into the garden, Maud,
>   For the black bat, night, has flown,
> Come into the garden, Maud,
>   I am here at the gate alone;
> And the woodbine spices are wafted abroad,
>   And the musk of the rose is blown.

It occurs to me that it is high honor for Tennyson to have his poetry quoted in heaven.

I turn, I twist, I twirl. I melt, I fade, I dissolve. No diaphanous cloud is so light and airy as I. I admire the ease with which I float. My gracefulness fills me with delight. My body is not subject to the law of gravitation. I sail dreamily along, lost in exquisite intoxication.

New scenes of wonder continually unravel themselves before my astonished eyes. I say to myself that if I could only record one one-thousandth of the ideas which come to me every second, I would be considered a greater poet than Milton.

I am on the top of a high mountain-peak. I am alone – only the romantic night envelops me. From a distant valley I hear the gentle tinkling of cow-bells. I float downwards, and find immense fields in which peacocks' tails are growing. They wave slowly, to better exhibit their dazzling ocelli, and I revel in the gorgeous colors. I pass over mountains and I sail over seas. I am the monarch of the air.

I hear the songs of women. Thousands of maidens pass near me, they bend their bodies in the most charming curves, and scatter beautiful flowers in my fragrant path. Some faces are strange, some I knew on earth, but all are lovely. They smile, and sing and dance. Their bare feet glorify the firmament. It is more than flesh can stand. I grow sensual unto satyriasis. The aphrodisiac effect is astonishing in its intensity. I enjoy all the women of the world. I pursue countless maidens through the confines of heaven. A delicious warmth suffuses my whole body. Hot and blissful I float through the universe, consumed with a resistless passion. And in the midst of this unexampled and unexpected orgy, I think of the case reported by the German Dr. Reidel, about a drug-clerk who took a huge dose of hasheesh to enjoy voluptuous visions, but who heard not even the rustle of Aphrodite's garment, and I laugh at him in scorn and derision.

I sigh deeply, open my eyes, and find myself sitting with one foot in bed, and the other on my desk. I am bathed in warm sweat which is pleasant. But my head aches, and there is a feeling in my stomach which I recognize and detest. It is nausea. I pull the basket near me, and await the inevitable result. At the same time I feel like begging for mercy, for I have traveled so far and so long, and I am tired beyond limit, and I need a rest. The fatal moment approaches, and I lower my head for the easier deposition of the rising burden. And my head seems monstrously huge, and weighted with lead. At last the deed is done, and I lean back on the pillow.

I hear my sister come home from the opera. I wish to call her. My sister's name is Ellen. I try to say it, but I cannot. The effort is too much. I sigh in despair. It occurs to me that I may achieve better results if I compromise on Nell, as this contains one syllable instead of two. Again I am defeated. I am too weary to exert myself to any extent, but I am determined. I make up my mind to collect all my strength, and call out: Nell. The result is a fizzle. No sound issues from my lips. My lips do not move. I give it up. My head falls on my breast, utterly exhausted and devoid of all energy.

Again my brain teems. Again I hear that high and heavenly harmony, again I float to the outposts of the universe and beyond, again I see the dancing maidens with their soft yielding bodies, white and warm. I am excited unto ecstasy. I feel myself a brother to the Oriental, for the same drug which gives him joy is now acting on me. I am conscious all the time, and I say to myself in a knowing way with a suspicion of a smile: All these visions because of 20 minims of Cannabis indica. My only regret is that the trances are ceaseless. I wish respite, but for answer I find myself floating over an immense ocean. Then the vision grows so wondrous, that body and soul I give myself up to it, and I taste the fabled joys of paradise. Ah, what this night is worth!

The music fades, the beauteous girls are gone, and I float no more. But the black rubber covering of my typewriter glows like a chunk of yellow phosphorus. By one door stands a skeleton with a luminous abdomen and brandishes a wooden sword. By the other door a little red devil keeps guard. I open my eyes wide, I close them right, but these spectres will not vanish. I know they are not real, I know I see them because I took hasheesh, but they annoy me nevertheless. I become uncomfortable, even frightened. I make a superhuman effort, and succeed in getting up and lighting the gas. It is two o'clock. Everything is the way it should be, except that in the basket I notice the remains of an orange – somewhat the worse for wear.

I feel relieved, and fall asleep. Something is handling me, and I start in fright. I open my eyes and see my father. He has returned from a meeting at the Academy of Medicine, and surprised at seeing a light in my room at such a time, has entered. He surmises what I have done, and is anxious to know what quantity I have taken. I should have answered, with a wink, *quantum sufficit*, but I have no inclination for conversation; on hearing the question repeated, I answer, "Twenty minims." He tells me I look as pale as a ghost, and brings me a glass of water. I drink it, become quite normal, and thus ends the most wonderful night of my existence.

In the morning my capacity for happiness is considerably increased. I have an excellent appetite, the coffee I sip is nectar, and the white bread ambrosia. I take my camera, and walk to Central Park. It is a glorious day. Everyone I meet is idealized. The lake never looked so placid before. I enter the hot-houses, and a gaudy-colored insect buzzing among the lovely flowers fills me with joy. I am too languid to take any pictures; to set the focus, to use the proper stop, to locate the image, to press the bulb – all these seem Herculean feats which I dare not even attempt. But I walk and walk, without apparent effort, and my mind eagerly dwells on the brilliant pageantry of the night before. I do not wish to forget my frenzied nocturnal revelry upon the vast dome of the broad blue heavens. I wish to remember forever, the floating, the mercury-globules, the peacock-feathers, the colors, the music, the women. In memory I enjoy the carnival all over again.

"For the brave Meiamoun," writes Theophile Gautier, "Cleopatra danced; she was apparelled in a robe of green, open at either side; castanets were attached to her alabaster hands.... Poised on the pink tips of her little feet, she approached swiftly to graze his forehead with a kiss; then she recommenced her wondrous art, and flitted around him, now backward-leaning, with head reversed, eyes half-closed, arms lifelessly relaxed, locks uncurled and loose – hanging like a bacchante of Mount Mænalus; now again active, animated, laughing, fluttering, more tireless and capricious in her movements than the pilfering bee. Heart-consuming love, sensual pleasure, burning passion, youth inexhaustible and ever-fresh, the promise of bliss to come – she expressed all…. The modest stars had ceased to contemplate the scene; their golden eyes could not endure such a spectacle; the heaven itself was blotted out, and a dome of flaming vapor covered the hall."

But for me a thousand Cleopatras caroused – and did not present me a vase of poison to drain at a draught. Again I repeated to myself: "And all these charming miracles because of 20 minims of *Fluidextractum Cannabis Indicæ*, U. S. P."

By the afternoon I had so far recovered as to be able to concentrate my mind on technical studies. I will not attempt to interpret my visions psychologically, but I wish to refer to one aspect. Spencer, in *Principles of Psychology*, mentions hasheesh as possessing the power of reviving ideas. I found this to be the case. I spoke about air-ships because there had been a discussion about them at supper; I quoted from Tennyson's *Maud* because I had been re-reading it; I saw mercury-globules in the heavens because that same day I had worked with mercury in preparing mercurial plaster; and I saw the peacock-tails because a couple of days previous I had been at the Museum of Natural History and had closely observed a magnificent specimen. I cannot account for the women.

All poets – with the possible exception of Margaret Sangster – have celebrated Alcohol, while Rudyard Kipling has gone so far as to solemnize delirium tremens; B. V. has glorified Nicotine; DeQuincey has immortalized Opium; Murger is full of praise for Caffeine; Dumas in *Monte Cristo* has apotheosized hasheesh, Gautier has vivified it in *Club des Hachicins*. Baudelaire has panegyrized it in *Artificial Paradises*, but as few American pens have done so, I have taken it upon myself to write a sonnet to the most interesting plant that blooms:

Near Punjab and Pab, in Sutlej and Sind,
Where the cobras-di-capello abound,
Where the poppy, palm and the tamarind,
With cummin and ginger festoon the ground –
And the capsicum fields are all abloom,
From the hills above to the vales below,
Entrancing the air with a rich perfume,
There too does the greenish Cannabis grow:
Inflaming the blood with the living fire,
Till the burning joys like the eagles rise,
And the pulses throb with a strange desire,
While passion awakes with a wild surprise: –
O to eat that drug, and to dream all day,
Of the maids that live by the Bengal Bay!

Appendix

MR. COURTENAY LEMON has written the following memorandum of the subjective features of his experience:

The first symptom which told me that the drug was beginning to take effect was a feeling of extreme lightness. I seemed to be hollowing out inside, in some magical manner, until I became a mere shell, ready to float away into space. This was soon succeeded, in one of the breathless intervals of my prodigious laughter, by a diametrically opposite sensation of extreme solidity and leaden weight. It seemed to me that I had changed into metal of some sort. There was a metallic taste in my mouth; in some inexplicable way the surfaces of my body seemed to communicate to my consciousness a metalliferous feeling; and I imagined that if struck I would give forth a metallic ring. This heavy and metallic feeling traveled rapidly upwards from the feet to the chest, where it stopped, leaving my head free for the issuance of the storms of laughter. Most of the time my arms and legs seemed to be so leaden that it required Herculean effort to move them, but under any special stimulus, such as the entrance of a third person, the vagrant conception of a new idea, or an unusually hearty fit of laughing, this feeling of unliftable heaviness in the limbs and torso would be forgotten and I would move freely, waving my arms with great vigor and enthusiasm.

Throughout the experiment I experienced a peculiar double consciousness. I was perfectly aware that my laughter, etc., was the result of having taken the drug, yet I was powerless to stop it, nor did I care to do so, for I enjoyed it as thoroughly as if it had arisen from natural causes. In the same way the extension of the sense of time induced by the drug was in itself indubitable and as cogent as any normal evidence of the senses, yet I remained able to convince myself at any moment by reflection that my sense of time was fallacious. I divided these impressions into hasheesh-time and real time. But in their alternations, so rapid as to seem simultaneous, both these standards of time seemed equally valid. For instance, once or twice when my friend spoke of something I had said a second before, I was impatient and replied: "What do you want to go back to that for? That was a long time ago. What's the use of going back into the past?" At the next moment, however, I would recognize, purely as a matter of logic, that he was replying to the sentence before the last that I had uttered, and would thus realize that the remark to which he referred was separated from the present only by a moment's interval. I did not, however, at any time on this occasion, attain the state sometimes reached in the second stage of hasheesh intoxication in which mere time disappears in an eternity wherein ages rush by like ephemera; nor did I experience any magnification of the sense of space, my experiences in regard to such extensions being confined to an intermittant multiplication of the sense of time.

When my laughter began it seemed for an instant to be mechanical, as if produced by some external power which forced air in and out of my lungs; it seemed for an instant to proceed from the body rather than from the mind; to be, in its inception, merely physical laughter without a corresponding psychic state of amusement. But this was only momentary. After the first few moments I enjoyed laughing immensely. I felt an inclination to joke as well as to laugh, and I remember saying: "I am going to have some reason for this laughing, so I will tell a story; if I have to laugh anyway, I'm going to supply good reasons for doing so, as it would be idiotic to laugh about nothing." I thereupon proceeded to relate an anecdote. Although I knew that my condition was the result of the drug, I was nevertheless filled with a genuine sense of profound hilarity, an eager desire to impart similar merriment to others, and a feeling of immense geniality and mirth, accompanied by sentiments of the most expansive good-will.

Against the effects of the drug, much as I enjoyed and yielded to it, there was opposed a preconceived intention. I had determined to tell my friend Victor Robinson, who was taking notes of my condition, just how I felt; had determined to supply as much data as possible in regard to my sensations. The result was that I repeatedly summoned all the rational energy that remained to me, and fought desperately to express the thoughts that came to me, whether ridiculous or analytical. Sometimes when I felt myself slipping away again into laughter or dreaminess I summoned all my strength to say what I had in mind, and would lose the thread of my thought and could not remember what I wanted to say, but would return to it again and again with the utmost determination and tenacity until I succeeded in saying what I wished to – sometimes an observation about my sensations, often only a jest about my condition. I believe that this acted as a great resistant to the effect of the drug. The energy of the drug was dissipated, I think, in overcoming my will to observe and analyze my sensations, and it was probably for this reason that I did not pass very far on this occasion into the second stage in which laughter gives place to grandiose visions and charming hallucinations.

After my friend Victor and his father turned out the light and left the room, my laughter gradually subsided into a few final gurgles of ineffable mirth and benevolence, and after a period of the amorous visions sometimes induced by this philtre from the land of harems, I fell into a sound sleep after my three hours of continuous and exhausting laughter.

I awoke next morning after seven hours sleep, with a ravenous appetite, which I think was probably as much due to the great expenditure of energy in laughing as to any direct effect of the drug itself. I was also very thirsty and my skin was parched and burning. Although I immediately dressed and went down to breakfast, I felt very drowsy and disinclined to physical exertion or mental concentration. And while no longer given to causeless laughter, I felt a lingering merriment and was easily moved to chuckling. I slept several hours in the afternoon and after dinner I slept all evening, awaking at 11 P. M., when I arose feeling very much refreshed and entirely normal, and went out to get another meal, being still hungry. I should say that the immediate after-effect, the reaction from the stimulation of hasheesh, is not much greater, except for the drowsiness, than that following the common or beer garden variety of intoxication. My memory of what I said and did while under the hasheesh was complete and accurate.

www.ingramcontent.com/pod-product-compliance
Lightning Source LLC
Chambersburg PA
CBHW051252170526
45165CB00004B/1682